Living Life
In Vitiligo

Living Life
In Vitiligo

Norene L. Willis

Library of Congress Control Number: 2008905053
ISBN: Hardcover   978-1-4363-4825-6
                 Softcover   978-1-4363-4824-9

To order additional copies of this book, contact:
Xlibris Corporation
1-888-795-4274
www.Xlibris.com
Orders@Xlibris.com
50022

Contents

To a world of people living in vitiligo, just like myself.

Acknowledgment

This book was written by the aid of the Holy Spirit, who daily leads and guides me to walk after Him. My prayer is for strength to follow His lead.

I want to thank my family for all their love and support for me during the time it took me to write this manuscript. God bless and keep each and every one of you.

I want to thank my husband, Mr. Garner R. Willis Sr., for having patience with me, for all of those weeks and months he spent alone entertaining himself. Honey, I love you. God bless you.

Honey, that was the icing on the cake when you called me on my job, expressing yourself about my book. That was the greatest.

Garner said, "Norene! You wrote a book. I did not know you had it in you. This is great. I was on page 13, and I had to stop and give you a call. I am so proud of you. This is very good. You explained everything to the people so that they would be able to understand it. I did not know that you had it in you! CONGRATULATIONS! GREAT JOB!"

Garner, you really know how to make a women feel great. It really meant a lot to me. I LOVE YOU, MAN!

To my daughter Teresa, who said, "I really like your book. It is very good. Great job, Mom."

To my daughter Arika, who told me, "This is really great. I know you were going to do a great job. I like it."

I also want to thank Arika so much for taking time out of her very busy schedule to type out my manuscript for me. I would not have been able to finish it without you. God bless you.

To my son Garner Jr. All he kept saying was, "I knew you could do it." You wrote it with love. It's reader friendly and very easy for people to understand.

To Amber, who said, "I really like this book. You explained everything where people can understand. Thanks so much for letting me read your book."

My prayer is that God our Father will bless you as you read this book, and that you will allow Jesus Christ to hold you ever so gently in His arms. To anoint you in His Holy Spirit, renew your mind, and give you a new heart with a faith the size of a mustard seed.

> *So Jesus said to them, "Because of your unbelief; for assuredly, I say to you. If you have faith as a mustard seed, you will say to this mountain, 'Move from here to there,' and it will move; and nothing will be impossible for you." (Matthew 17:20)*

That you will never be the same again and that you will live out your life the way in which God ordained you to live from the beginning of creation. In Christ Jesus's name, Amen.

God bless you,

Norene Lezette Willis

A short preview of what's to come: There are about two MILLION people who are affected with this vitiligo worldwide.

My name is Norene Lezette Willis. I was born in Marion, Indiana, on April 28, 1943. Yes, I am a country girl and proud of it. I am the fourth child in my family. My mom had eight children.

My mother had a brother who had vitiligo. As a child, this was the only way I ever remembered seeing him. I never paid too much attention to it. By the time I reached my twenty-third birthday, I too started to get patches of silver hair on my head. I still did not know at the time that it was the beginning stages of vitiligo. During that time I did not want anyone to know I had gray hair. So I would comb my hair in such a way that nobody would ever know I had gray hair. For years this went on until streaks in one's hair became fashionable and ladies started to frost their hair. Then I started to comb my hair so that people could see my gray hair. I started to get compliments, and I liked that. So finally this gave me encouragement to adjust to my silver hair.

It seems as if things happen in cycles of every ten years. One morning I woke up, I was just looking in the mirror, when I realized that my lips were white. Just like that, overnight! My gums used to be a very dark brown, now they too were pink. That morning my son asked me, "When did your lips turn white?" Overnight, Son! Then my hands started to get whites patches too. This was the hardest thing for me to get used to. I just did not recognize my hands. The children everywhere I went were afraid to touch or shake my hands. They would ask, "Why are your hands dirty?" Or they would say, "Look at your hands!" They would start to point and stare. Then their lower lips would drop down, and their eyes would fasten directly on my hands. Sometimes they would not speak, but just tug on their parent's clothes to get their attention. Most of the time the parent's response would be, "Oh, she was born like that," or they would just turn and walk the other way to keep from answering their questions.

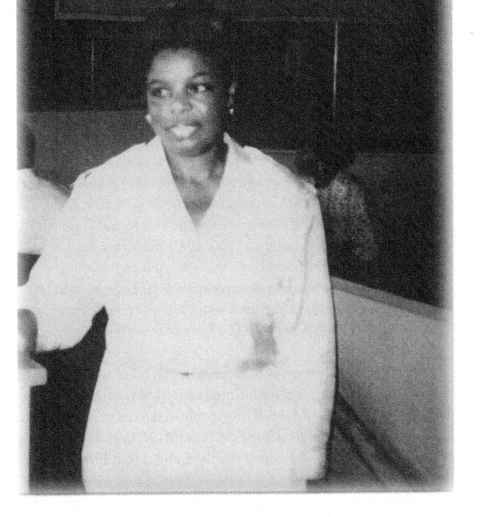

The truth of the matter was, I really did not mind the kids asking me questions. I would rather talk to them directly, than have them stare and wonder. The parents though think that they were embarrassing me, but they were not. What you do not understanding is when you ask questions then we both feel better.

By now, my cheeks and around my eyes were white. I still never went to the doctor, because I thought it was hereditary and there was nothing that could be done about it. One day, my cousin and his wife came to visit us from Washington DC. His wife said to me that there was a cure for vitiligo. This was the first time I actually found out what the name of this illness was.

I used to think it was leprosy, a common disease in the Bible.

> *When the leprous sore is on a person, then he shall be brought to the priest. And the priest shall examine him; and indeed if the swelling on the skin is white, and it has turned the hair white, and there is a spot of raw flesh in the swelling, it is an old leprosy on the skin of his body. The priest shall pronounce him unclean, and shall not isolate him, for he is unclean. And if leprosy breaks out all over the skin, and the leprosy covers all the skin of the one who has the sore, from his head to his foot, wherever the priest looks, then the priest shall consider; and indeed if the leprosy has covered all his body, he shall pronounce him clean who has the sore. It has all turned white. He is clean. (Leviticus 13:9-13)*

But I knew that leprosy were sores, and that is not what I have; but I felt as if it was what I had each time I heard the pastor talk about it in his sermons, and I felt as if all the people in the church thought that this was what was wrong with me. So I would just keep silent, waiting for the feeling to go away. Some people thought that I had been in a fire and had been burned.

Eventually I did go to a doctor, who said that the cause of my illness was vitiligo. My white blood cells have the tendency to destroy themselves. This is what causes the pigment to be lacking in my complexion and the patches to appear. I talked to my husband about going to a doctor to find out more about it. But he did not want me to do anything about it. But it was my face!

In the meantime, I spoke to a coworker. I was looking for a second opinion regarding my diagnosis. She encouraged me to go and find out more about it, then make my decisions later. I called the doctor, made an appointment, and went in to see him. He suggested I go to Boston to see a specialist. This is where I met all kinds of people who looked just like I did. There were all races of people there going through the exact same illness. That is when I realized that I was not alone. There are white people turning black and black people turning white. Admittedly, it was scary to see so many people at one time. We are all at different stages and degrees of this vitiligo. Some people are just starting out, while others have been going through it for some time. But we are all in this together. That day in the doctor's office, I knew then that we needed each other.

That our hearts needed to be encouraged, being kitted together in love. (Colossians 2:2b)

The doctor told me then that there is no cure for this illness, but it is treatable. The treatment was called blue florescent lighting. It is artificial lighting being treated with an ointment to activate the pigment in your body to cause the tone to return to normal. First thing, you are placed in this tub for a few seconds at a time. As your treatment progresses, your minutes increase until your complexion starts to get its pigment back. After your treatment, you have to put on ointment to protect yourself from the sun's rays. It is also essential to wear sunglasses, a wide brim hat, and long sleeves to protect you from the sun's natural rays.

In the meantime, I started to research this vitiligo:

It is thought to be an autoimmune disorder, in which the body produces antibodies that react against its own tissues. The antibodies destroy the cells in the skin that produces melanin. Typically, about one in three people with vitiligo have a family history of this condition. Treatment is typically ultraviolet (UV) light phototherapy or drug called psoralen. This increases the sensitivity of the skin to light. This treatment usually used for psoralen is called PUVA (psoralen and ultraviolet light). The outcome: pigmented patches continue to enlarge slowly.

Vitiligo: Characterized by patches of white skin due to loss of normal pigment (melanin) from patches of skin. Most commonly occurring on the face and hands, vitiligo is more obvious in people with dark skin.

Melanin: A brownish-black pigment found in the skin, hair, etc., (from the Greek term *melas*, meaning "black"). Autoimmune disorder is the cause.

Auto: A. Combining form meaning (1) self, (2) by one's self or itself (from the Greek word *autos*, meaning "self").

Immune: Without *munia*, duties. Exempt from or protected against something disagreeable or harmful. Not susceptible to a specified disease.

I have been receiving treatment for two years now. The patches on my face did get better, but it did not come back in my natural skin tone—it was much darker. This ended my treatment for now. Well, by the grace of God, I have been able to adjust to this condition, and thank God that this illness or condition will not take my life.

Ten years later, this vitiligo came back on me again. When I returned to the doctor's office, they told me then that Blue Cross Blue Shield were no longer covering this treatment under their policy; it was now considered cosmetic surgery. That is when the doctor introduced me to Dermablend makeup with a powder base. It is sold in the local department stores. At first, I liked the makeup. It covered well; people did not know I even had it on. I was getting great compliments at both church and at work. I would wear it everywhere I went. I would not leave the house without it. There were times when I returned home from shopping and had already removed my makeup, only to realize that I had forgotten something to complete my dinner that night. Needless to say, I was not going back out for anything.

There was a time when my daughter came over after church with her boyfriend, and I was unaware he was with her until he was walking up the stairs. All I could think of was him going back to the church and telling the congregation about my vitiligo. He did not, but this was what I was thinking.

It has been five years now since I have been wearing this Dermablend, and I was tired of getting it all over my clothes. The instructions said that it is supposed to stay in place, but that was not the case. It turned out that everybody I hugged was wearing my makeup too. I spoke to everybody, and I hugged on everybody. God has given me the gift to hug people, and now the makeup was getting in the way. But deep down on the inside, I knew that this was not the real me. I felt that one day, this makeup would have to go.

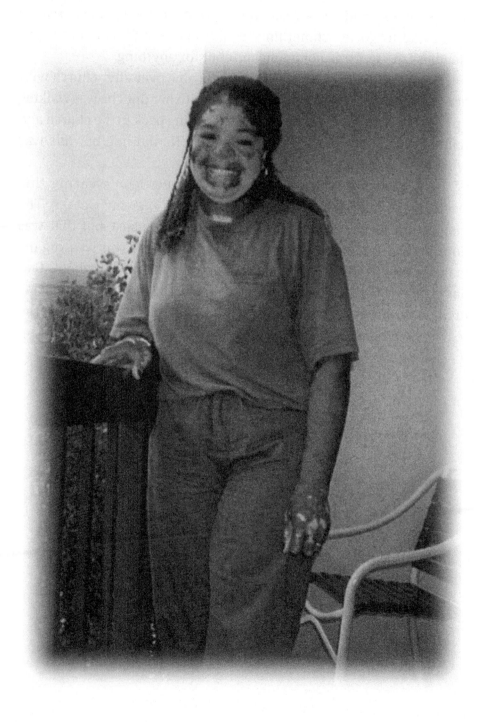

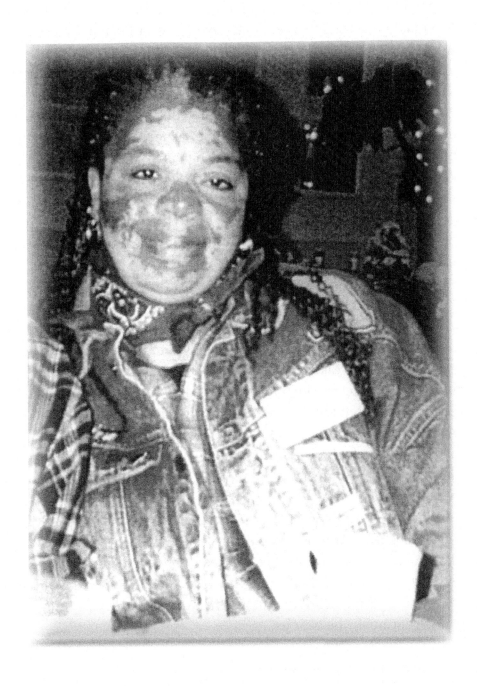

I had been a member of the church for a few years now. I sang in the choir, but I kept to myself a lot. This was a much bigger church than I had been used to attending. Have you ever been in a crowd of people but you felt as if you were all alone?

About thirteen years ago, I was invited to attend a women's retreat in Sharon, Massachusetts, held by the women at Morning Star Baptist Church in Mattapan, Massachusetts. I had never been on a women's retreat before, so I did not know what to expect to get out of it. One thing I did know was that I needed a change in my life. The women who went to these retreats had already picked out their roommate in advance, but I did not know the women enough to choose a roommate. So I went alone. When I got there, they had already picked out a roommate for me. Her name was Cynthia. I did not know her, but ever since that day, we have been the best of friends.

The name of their theme was "Taking Off the Mask." There were about a hundred women there. We all were gathered together in the auditorium. They had formed a prayer line, and one by one each of us were prayed over and anointed with oil. When it became my turn, I knew that I had to take the makeup off because the Lord had already laid it upon my heart. The minister prayed for me, and I let her know then that I wanted to take the makeup off, but I really did not know what the outcome was going to be. There were two other ladies at the retreat who had gone through some major surgery of their own. They each had volunteered to assist me to my room and wait for me to remove my makeup.

When we returned to the auditorium, Minister Spence said, "Oh you are beautiful. Your face is glowing. There is an aura around you." The women in the retreat were all great. They all rallied around me with love and compassion in their hearts, and we all prayed that God would heal all our fears and deliver us, that a hedge of protection would continually be over us.

He is a shield to all who trust in him.

(II Samuel 22:31b)

We all prayed for one another for unity, for the love and strength, for faith that God would see us through.

Trust in the Lord with all your heart and lean not unto your own understanding.

(Proverbs 3:5)

And my God shall supply all your needs. According to His riches in Glory by Christ Jesus.

(Philippians 4:19)

I will lift up mine eyes unto the hills from which cometh your help

(Psalm 121:1)

Minister Spence told me then that God had picked me out to be picked on. On Sunday morning before we departed to go our own separated ways, we all gathered together in a huge circle in the parking lot. We were all arm and arm, taking turns praying for one another. They all made a vow then that they would be a support chain for me and keep in touch with me, for as long as I needed them. We all need to hold on to our faith that has kept us all these years. God will see us through.

For we walk by faith not by sight. (II Corinthians 5:7)

Standing On The Promises Of God Standing On His Word

It has been a lifetime journey, but god is my savior:
I can do all things through Christ who strengthens me.
—Philippians 4:13

As a child, I was totally withdrawn. I was a very shy person. I used to stutter when I talked. I was dying to speak but when it became my turn to talk I would lose my thought.

The teacher pushed my desk right up against her desk, so that she could hear what I had to say. I was talking barely above a whisper. Nobody even knew I was there. After I got married, I was slowly coming out of it. It has been years since this happened to me, and I have been running to catch up with all of what I lost out on when I was a child. But now, I felt it coming back on me again.

It was in November 1996 when I first started this walk. It was the Lord and I. This is the only way any of us will be able to make it thus far. I recall the Sunday when I drove home from Sharon, Massachusetts. With out my makeup on. I knew in my heart that God was right there with me. When I arrived home, my husband asked me, "Where are you coming from without your makeup on?" Now he knew I was at the retreat all weekend, but he was so surprised to see me coming in the house without my makeup on. But he was cool. He has always told me that I did not need the makeup and that he would always be there for me through thick and thin, and that we would go through it together, for better or worst.

Early the next morning, my telephone started to ring. It was one of the ladies from the retreat. She called me and asked me how I was doing. She started to pour into me words of encouragement. She told me that I was a very brave woman and that she would be there for me. She gave me her phone numbers and told me to call her any time of the day, at her home or in her office. She ensured me that she would be there for me. She then began to pray for me. I thanked her so much for calling me the first thing in the morning. Right after that call, another woman called me and told me that she was very proud of me and that this was a great step of faith for me, and she blessed me and prayed for me. This went on for weeks at a time; one woman after another was calling me, praying with me, crying with me, pouring into me, giving me words of wisdom, telling me to hold my head up.

> *For He Himself has said, "I will never leave you nor forsake you." (Hebrews 13:5B)*

> *So we may boldly say, "The Lord is my helper; I will not fear. What can man do to me?" (Hebrews 13: 6)*

Several women called me in the morning. But Minister Dotty Smith called me before I got up in the morning and told me that she wanted to pray with me before I get out of my bed, before I start my day.

God is such a good god! He will place godly people all around you. God and all of His angels will lift you up and carry you. When you are too fragile, He will make you strong.

> *Therefore humble yourselves under the mighty hand of God, that He may exalt you in due time. Casting all your cares upon Him, for He cares for you.*
>
> *(I Peter 5:6-7)*

On that following Monday morning when I arrived for work, my boss said to me, "What is this, we are not used to this!" Meaning that I was not wearing my makeup. I said to him, "Neither am I!"

I am adjusting to my coworkers while they are adjusting to me. It is all a process. We are going to need the patience of Job. But remember one thing, if God has brought you to it, He will bring you through it.

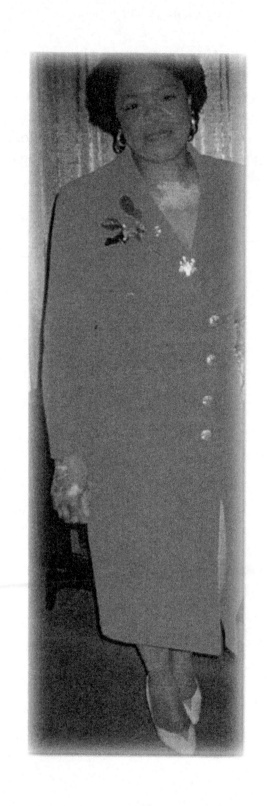

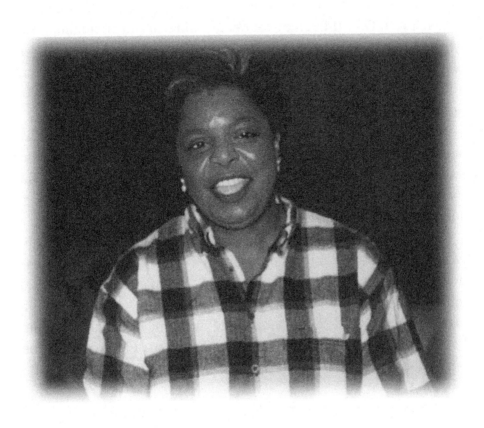

Over the course of several weeks, I received six to eight phone calls a day from the women of God. On Sunday morning when I came to church, the people showed such love. Everybody was so compassionate, warm, and friendly toward me. There were men and women who came up to me and said, "You are beautiful just the way you are."

There is one thing I would like to make very clear. There are people who will not like you, who think you have a disease, and who are afraid to touch you. They think that your condition will rub off on them. You will meet people who will ask you if you are "white turning black or black turning white." We have been picked out to be picked on. We are going to go through some stuff. This will take some time. Vitiligo did not just happen overnight.

We are lumps of coal—totally unpolished, rough on all sides. God is just chipping away on the outside edges of our souls. God is not finished with us, yet one day we all will come forth as pure gold. But today, we are being tried through the fire. All of us are going through something—some more than others.

In the beginning, I hated to look in the mirror at myself. I did whatever I had to do and got out from in front of the mirror. You see, I do not have to look at myself—you do. In the Bible, it says after a man looks at himself in the mirror, he soon forgets what he looks like. That is why when people stare at me, I forget what my face looks like, until I see the expression on their faces. It then causes me to remember what I look like.

> For if any one is a hearer of the word and not a doer, he is like a man observing his natural face in a mirror. For he observes himself, goes away and immediately forgets what kind of man he was. (James1:23-24)

One day around Halloween time, there was a complete stranger who asked me, "What are you supposed to be?" I said, "What?" At first, I did not know what he was talking about, but then I remembered he was talking about my face. I just turned and kept walking.

One day, you will feel as if you are a sideshow and you have not even scratched the surface yet. So do whatever you have to do and get out of the mirror. We cannot do anything on our own. It is Jesus. It is all about Jesus, and none of you. God promised to fight our battles.

> *And all this assembly shall know that the Lord saveth not with sword and spear; for the battle is the Lord's and He will give you into our hands. (I Samuel 17:47)*

After Vitiligo
We All Shall Live Again

We must pour into ourselves words of encouragement. To learn to love yourself, to take time out for yourselves. Learn to look in the mirror at yourself. Tell yourself how much you love yourself. Tell yourself how great you look. Build yourself up; speak over yourself words of wisdom and acknowledgment. The Bible tells us to "prophesy over yourself. To call those things that are not, as though they are."

> I will praise you, for I am fearfully and wonderfully made;
> Marvelous are Your work, and that my soul knows very well.
> (Psalm 139:1)

> For we know in part and we prophesy in part. But when that
> which is perfect is come then that which is in part shall be done
> away with. (I Corinthians 13:9-10)

> Now faith is the substance of things hoped for, the evidence of
> things not seen. (Hebrew 11:1)

So, people, take a real good look at yourself from the inside out. Learn to love yourself. Pull yourself up by your own bootstraps and say to yourself, "I can make it, one day at a time!" I can do all things through Christ who strengths me. I am somebody!

God is taking us all somewhere. He has a great service for all of us to do. I'm a gospel singer in my church, and I also sing with the praise and worship team. I am up on stage all of the time, and there are people trying to intimidate me, trying to make me feel self-conscious, and distracting me to make me feel uneasy about myself. God is making me stronger every day. If looks could kill, we would all be dead.

I used to allow the devil to dictate to me. He would say to me, "They do not like your singing. Look at you." But I tell you right now, do not allow your mind to even toy with the devil! Shut him down the moment he starts to raise his ugly head. Be firm and direct. If you have to, shout it out! If you have to, stomp your feet! But get your point across loud and clear. Change the subject in your mind, stay positive, and look for the good in people and things around you. Say to yourself, I am somebody!

The Bible tells us to,

> *Set your mind on things above, and not on things on the earth. (Colossians 3:2)*

The Bible tells to

> *Finally, brethren, whatsoever things are true, whatever things are noble, whatsoever things are: "just whatever things are lovely. Whatsoever things are of good report, if there is any virtue and if there is any thing praiseworthy, meditate on these things. The things which you learned and received and heard and saw in me. These do, and "the God of peace will be with you." (Philippians 4:8-9)*

> *Be anxious for nothing, but in everything by prayer and supplication, with thanksgiving, let your requests be made known to God. (Philippians 4:6)*

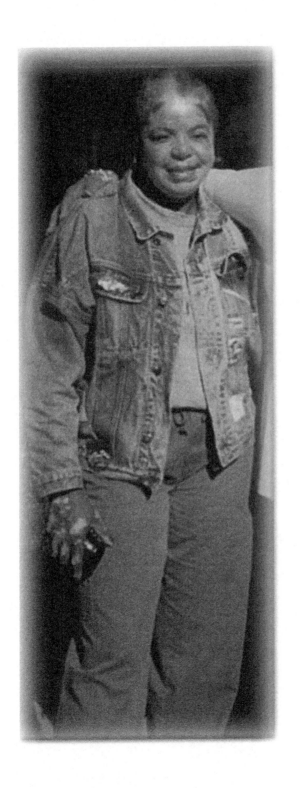

"Praise The Lord,
For He Is Good!"

Keep your faith, stay positive, and learn to pray no matter where you're at—on your feet, on your back, or on your knees. The devil is a liar, and his playground is in your mind. God dwells in your heart. Let your heart be your guide. In due time, God will strengthen your heart.

> *You are of God, little children, and have overcome them, because He who is in you is greater than he who is in the world. (I John 4:4)*

God's been very good to you. You must learn not to waste time worrying about things you have no control over.

It's all Jesus and none of you. We all must stay prayed up and ready at all times.

The Bible tells us

> *But sanctify the Lord God in our hearts: and be ready at all times to give an answer to every man that asketh you a reason of the hope that is in you with meekness and fear. (I Peter 3:15)*

It has been thirteen years now since I have stopped wearing that makeup, and I can do all things through Christ Jesus who strengthens me. God will keep you, and when you fall short, get back up again and keep on going, because there are too many people hurting. We all need to hold on to God's unchanging hand. Reach up and grab a hold of God.

> *I can do all things through Christ who strengtheneth me. (Philippians 4:13)*

We all have a job to do. There is a world of vitiligo people out there, which are hiding behind closed doors, under makeup, behind sunglasses and wide-brimmed hats, behind loved ones, and away from their enemies. People are too afraid to step out, to go on with their lives, because of what they look like or in fear of what people will say about them.

> *For God has not given us a spirit of fear, but of power and of love and of a sound mind. (II Timothy 1:7)*

I am a living testimony; we all are living testimonies. There is a whole town of people in Plymouth who do not know who I am, because of my vitiligo. But I have to go on; you have to go on and get on with your life! God made you just the way you are, and the Bible says that we are fearfully and wonderfully made.

You see, I love myself very much. Yes, I wish that I did not have vitiligo, but there is nothing that I can do about it. There is nothing that you can do about it. So get on with your life.

I keep pictures of myself all around my home before vitiligo and after vitiligo. I get in the mirror and just talk to myself. I am always talking to myself. "Hey, Reenie! How you be badobazin? I love you. You got it going on, girl!" "You men you must go on there's no turning back". I will go right up to the mirror and kiss myself in the mirror. No, I did not say that I did not have anybody around me to kiss me. I said that is me, myself, and I motivating myself. I am building myself up for me and me alone. I have decided a long time ago that this is my life. I am not coming this way again. I have one chance to live out my life in Jesus's name. You have only one chance to live out your life, so get up, get going, start living again. We are only coming this way once.

Do Not Waste It Away! There Is No Coming Back. So Look Out World, Because Here I Commmmmmmme!

The Lord is my light and my salvation; whom shall I fear? The Lord is the strength of my life, of whom shall I be afraid? When the wicked came against me to eat up my flesh, my enemies and foes stumbled and fell. Though an army may encamp against me, my heart shall not fear: though war may rise against me, in this will I be confident. One thing have I desired of the Lord, that will I seek: that I may dwell in the house of the Lord all the days of my life, to behold the beauty of the Lord, and to enquire in his temple. For in the time of trouble he shall hide me in his pavilion: in the secret place of his tabernacle he shall hide me. He shall set me high upon a rock. And now my head shall be lifted up above my enemies all around me. Therefore will I offer sacrifices of joy in His tabernacle; I will sing, yea, I will sing praises unto the Lord. (Psalm 27:1-6)

Today. This day. I am going to live my life out even if it kills you. Why do I say that? Some people love misery. They love to put you down, to get you mad, to hurt your feelings, to just stir up trouble. But you have to rise above all that stuff. Look on the right side of things and keep on smiling. Look at it this way: it could have been terminal cancer. It could have been AIDS. It could have been a lot of things, but it is vitiligo. It will not kill you.

Years ago, I used to kid around with my husband that he will have the best of two worlds—the first half with a black woman and the second half with a white woman.

At one time, I used to feel sorry for myself and for my family, because this did not only happened to me, but it happened to my whole family also. Yes, I am the one with vitiligo, but the after effects go deeper and wider than one can imagine. It goes across the board—from my husband, my children, and my grandchildren, my church family.

I asked my children how they felt about this vitiligo, and they said to me, "What vitiligo? I do not see it. We see you, Mamma, and we love you." My husband loves me very much. We all at one time have wished life to be different. But it is not about you, it is all about Jesus and none of you. So go ahead and live out your life to the fullest. My family is always trying to protect me or defending me from what people are saying out loud or what they are saying to my face, or behind my back. Many times, I am walking two steps behind my husband, subconsciously wanting him to shield me. We all are going to go through some things. Remember this one thing, you're already in a storm, or you have just came out of a storm. These are all trials, and each time it will be a greater level than the first one. God is preparing us, getting us ready for His purpose, not yours. It is all about Him and none of you.

> *Jesus promise, for He Himself has said, "I will never leave you nor forsake you thee will always be there for us" So we may boldly say, "The Lord is my helper: I will not fear: What can man do to me? (Hebrews 13b:5-6)*

The Bible said

Trust in the Lord with all your heart: and lean not unto your own understanding. (Proverbs 3:5)

While we look not at the things which are seen, but at the things which are not seen: for all things which are seen are temporal; but the things which are not seen are eternal. (II Corinthians 4:18)

For we walk by faith, not by sight. (II Corinthians 5:7)

For we are saved by hope: but hope that is seen is not hope: for what a man seeth, why doth he yet hope for? But if we hope for that we see not, then do we with patience wait for it. (Romans 8:24, 25)

This is your life. Whatever has been dealt to you, God will give you the strength and the courage to live it out. Be yourself. You have gifts and talents. Use them for the glory of God, or you will lose them to someone else who is worse off than you.

I walk a lot, and I am always speaking to people everywhere I go. It has happened twice to me, by two different women who do not know each other, but they each said to me that the reason I speak to so many people is that this is a way of distracting people from staring at my vitiligo. I never thought of it that way because I am from Indiana, and back there, this is what we do: we speak to every body, and no one is considered a stranger. But I am in New England now, and they do things a little differently. They speak only if they know you. My attitude is, maybe it is time to change. People are people all over the world.

You will always be drawn to other people with vitiligo, because of what you have been through. We will always need the comfort from each other. I have learned to go right up to those people, introduce myself, and talk to them. Before we depart, I feel the need to just love on them—and I am not talking about a quick hug, and I am out of there. I am talking about holding on to each other, just for a little while, to give them some LOVE. You will get LOVE back in return. You see, God has given me the gift to hug people. That is just what I do. You have to be yourself despite yourself.

After all these years, people still come up to me in church and on my job and continue to ask me, "How are you?" Each time, the answer is "I am fine," because one day sooner or later, I will be fine.

> *Now faith is the substance of things hoped for, the evidence of things not seen. (Hebrews 11:1)*

They tell me that I am a testimony. My responses to that is, so are you. All of us are testimonies. God has blessed us to be a blessing to somebody else. It should never be all of me and none of you. Give it away! There is another blessing waiting for you. Look up! It is right above your head! Reach up and grab it down; it is your blessing. Just make up in your mind that you are going to live life to the fullest. Step out on your faith. It actually feels wonderful.

Now it is time for you to get back everything the devil has stolen from you. Your joy, your pride, your happiness, your peace of mind, your self-esteem—YOU.

> *And the peace of God, which surpasses all understanding, will guard your Hearts and minds through Christ Jesus. (Philippians 4:7)*

You are going to get back to being yourself again! It is time for you to allow yourself to live again. Go ahead, go out to dinner with your husband, your wife, your loved ones, your best friends, your old friends. Get back to life! God wants you to be whole. Remember this one thing, when you are in Jesus, you are never alone. Give it all to Jesus, and He will reward you eternally. Go ahead, go back to church, go to the mall, take that walk that you used to take months or even years ago. Get back to jogging again or riding that brand-new bike that has been collecting dust. Let your hair down, and allow it to blow in the wind. Learn to laugh at yourself or just sit on your porch, swinging in your swing, listening to nature's sounds in the woods, or just watching stars twinkling in the cool of the evening. It is time to be you, so snuggle up next to that special someone and just enjoy life. Learn how to grow old together. Stop wasting time and your life away.

> *Take therefore no thought for the tomorrow: for tomorrow shall take thought for the things of itself. Sufficient unto the day is the evil thereof. (Matthew 6:34)*

Tomorrow is not promised to any of us. Your life was brought and paid for by Jesus Christ on the cross at Calvary. The shedding of His precious blood. When He became the sacrificial lamb for our sins. We all have a debt to pay. Do you know that your testimony will win souls to the Lord? Being a witness to someone else who is struggling just like you. Our reward is ETERNAL. Remember?

We Have Been Picked Out To Be Picked On

"For I will restore health to you and heal you of your wounds," *says the Lord. "Because they called you an outcast saying, 'This* *is Zion, no one seeks her.'" (Jeremiah 30:17)*

For God so loved the world, that He gave His only begotten Son, *that whosoever believeth in Him should not perish, but have* *everlasting life. (John 3:15-16)*

Search the scriptures, find out what your purpose is in life, and get started. There is a world of people dying every day, wishing that their illness were vitiligo, rather than some deadly disease, and not on a countdown. One more thing to keep in mind: true beauty is on the inside, so allow it to

SHINE THROUGH YOU!

What are you waiting for? Step out into the sunlight and shine!

I have had vitiligo ever since I was twenty-three years old. I am now sixty-five years old.

It has been forty-two years. What would have happened if I just curled up and died forty-two years ago? I'm living life to the fullest.

Every time you see me, I am going to have a smile on my face, because this is only a

TEST OF MY FAITH!

GOD BLESS YOU, IN JESUS'S NAME.